# INTRODUCTION

Our makeup blog started primarily from my beautiful wife Shannon's love for everything makeup and cosmetics. I'm definitely a bit of an entrepreneur by heart and I'm always looking for neat new projects and business ideas to pursue. I came up with the concept of MakeupFOMO, at least a very watered down idea for the concept, and when I pitched it to Shannon her response was definitely lukewarm at best.

Once I put together a cheap and simply blog that actually put the idea into practice so she could see it live on a page, she really warmed up to it. Over the course of the next two years we've continuously changes our process for content creation, what the site is about, what it looks like, all of these things have changed drastically over time. At this point it's hard for me to even point to a place in time where I feel that THIS is where MakeupFOMO in its truest form started.

The success we have reached now is very comfortable. We get a great stream of traffic that earns us a comfortable amount of money consistently each month. The beauty of it is that the amount of "work" that goes into the site has stayed pretty consistent over time. Typically we each spend a few hours each week. The amount of money we make has drastically increased, over the same amount of work.

This book is based on the experience we've had in starting the blog and growing it to a successful and profitable venture. We have a lot ahead of us and tons of opportunity. Throughout this ebook I detail the strategies and approaches that we took to get our blog to this wonderful point.

# THE ROAD AHEAD

Creating a Makeup or Beauty blog is one of the most exciting things you can decide to do. If you've reached this point then this is probably an idea that you've been thinking about for quite some time. Most people realize that these days being a Makeup Guru or Beauty Influencer is a highly sought after job. These individuals who have propelled themselves to this status are able to amass huge sums of money and free products simply by doing what they love, which is talking/writing about makeup and beauty! What an envious position that truly is. It is not uncommon for beauty bloggers to make in excess of $5,000-$15,000 a month, with paid promotional events, paid vacations, etc. We've definitely all looked at this situation and thought to ourselves.. I could do this. Why don't I start blogging? I would love a job where I can write about my passion and replace my full time income! I could work from anywhere, and be one of those travelling gurus that you always see on a beach in Bora Bora...

So here is where I try to lay out the ground work of what is in front of you before you begin this journey. The road ahead is very tough, and it is littered with young men and women who drive themselves crazy trying to get to the position described above. What you are marveling at with these amazing beauty gurus is the product of a combination of luck and/or persistence. It is very common for the most popular bloggers to be individuals who have been doing this for many years. What's more is that they did not begin to see even a small amount of that success until very late in the game. I've seen the stats of many successful bloggers and they did not make any legitimate amount of money until they were at least 3-5 years into it, with consistent hard work all along the way. This is the reality of what creating a successful blogging empire looks like. This eBook will get you up and running and get you the tools and strategies needed to get you down the road successfully, but it is up to you to find the passion and dedication to consistently push forward when the going gets tough. And trust me... the going will get tough. So buckle down and get ready to head down this fantastic journey in one of the most amazing blogging opportunities currently available.

# GETTING STARTED

## *To be Frugal or Not? What's your budget?*

So now you've decided you're really going to do this! You're going to hop into the blogging world! But where do you begin? Well let's look at the high level decisions you need to make first. You need to decide if you are going to take the frugal approach, or if you just want to jump head first into this from the beginning. The frugal approach means that you will attempt to spend as little money as possible and only begin spending money on the blog once you feel you are ready to head into those latter stages. Jumping head first is.. well just that! Pretty much this means that you'll go right past some of the initial stages and move into the more advanced tools which require that you start spending money, in most cases this can average between \$20-\$50 in initial startup costs, and then around \$5-\$20 a month for various other services.

Our approach was to do the frugal method and this is typically what I would recommend to anyone approaching a new venture like this. The reason being is that when you are first starting out, you may not have a complete vision of what your blog will be, what the content will be like, how your approach to blogging will be. These are the types of questions that will typically be answered simply through doing. You need to get your hands dirty and start writing and creating in order to truly find your voice and what you enjoy doing. With that comes many of the small decisions you'll need to make regarding your blog. Therefore, if you know that you will likely change your mind many times, or if you aren't entirely sure on whether blogging is truly for you, then the frugal approach is probably for you. Why commit a bunch of money while you're still figuring it all out? In my opinion there is no need to rush into the paid services and advanced features before you're ready, you really don't miss out on a lot in the beginning. Our frugal approach sets you up with the important must-haves from Day 1, but the other advanced tools are really the icing on the cake that will set you up for the long haul. Let's layer that on once you're good and ready.

On the other hand, some people may have a very clear idea of what they want our of their blog and a solid vision for their content. If you're one of these people, well you're already off to a great start in which case you may decide to move past some of the early steps that we recommend. We do however, recommend that you at least read those sections. Many of the approaches we recommend are done for specific reasons. I'd suggest that you read those sections with an eye towards the big picture "why" are we doing these activities, and see how you can apply the same why to your own approach to the blog. I will try my best to lay it all out and explain my thinking behind it all and where it got us in the long run.

## Step 1: Welcome your blog into the world

As you may have guessed, the first step is to create your blog. Now you may think to yourself, what if I don't have a name yet?! Well I'm going to assume that you're going to use this as an opportunity to ponder this carefully. However, thankfully here in the beginning things are very fluid. You are more than welcome to change your mind which is the beauty of this approach. Many times the best way to know what you don't like, is to actually see it live on the screen. So create something, then keep an open mind to how you can improve or change it all together.

To begin we suggest (for the frugal approach) to create your blog on one of that many free blogging platforms. We definitely suggest and heavily favor that you do so on Wordpress.com. The reason being is that the Wordpress blogging platform is one of the most robust and popular platforms on the internet. The amount of guides, tools, and general "stuff" available for the Wordpress platform is just incredible. Above all else, the platform itself is free to use which I think is an important point because you don't want to get bled dry of money while you wait patiently for your blog to become a mega success. Also Wordpress.com has a super easy transition to Wordpress.org which is the advanced more robust blogging platform that you can host with a much more sophisticated web host. So my recommendation is absolutely Wordpress.com.

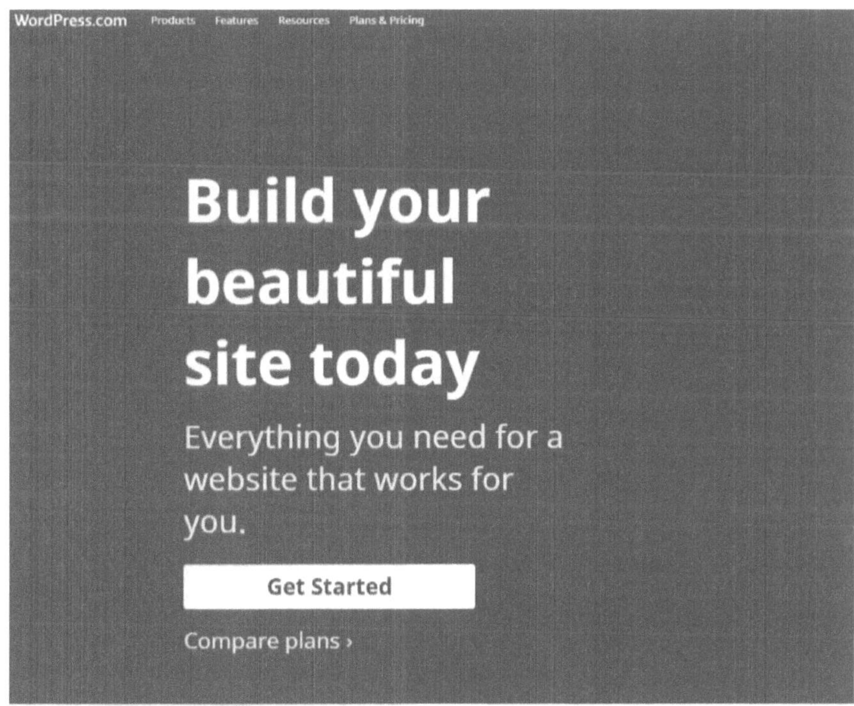


When you start your blog you'll be presented with the various plans that Wordpress.com has available. The way Wordpress.com works is that they are a paid host, meaning that they install the Wordpress blogging platform and manage the actual website and server and all you have to worry about is creating the content. The reason they do this is because they hope that you will keep using them and upgrade to their other paid packages to get a bunch of awesome features. We will not recommend that you do that. What we recommend is that when the time is right, you have a much cheaper and more reliable webhost manage the server and blogging platform, but enough on that later.

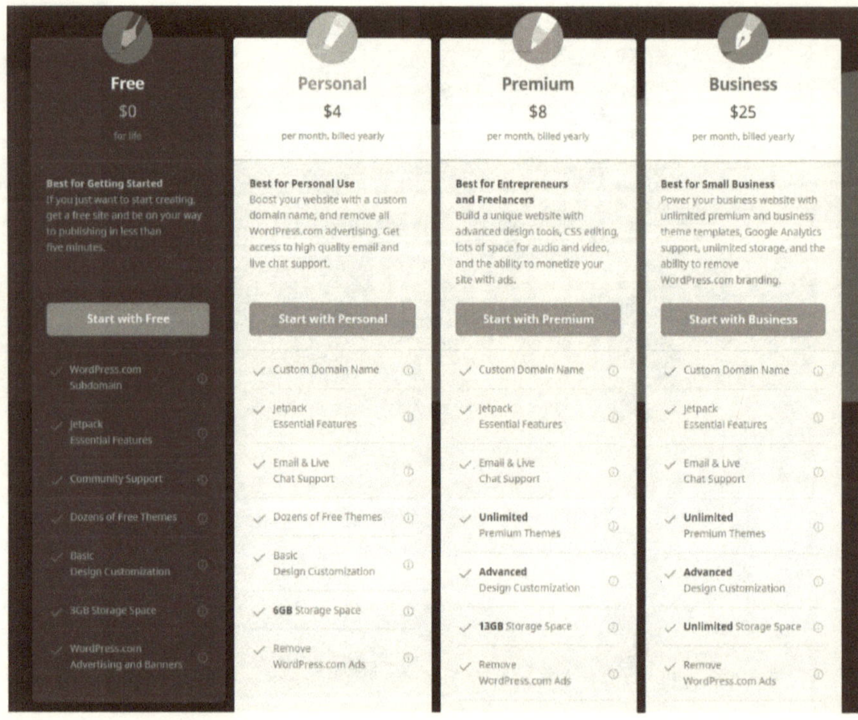


You're going to start with the Free version to begin. As you can see in the packaging layout this comes with all the features you need to create a Wordpress blog with a basic theme, do some basic customization, but overall we are just trying to get something created so that we can begin to tweak and allow you to find your voice in the type of content you want to create.

## Let's create a site.



Go ahead and move through the steps on the screen, and I'll meet you on the other side to go through the important pieces of what comes next. Right off the bat, Wordpress.com will try to talk you into moving into their paid plan and purchase a custom domain for your blog. My recommendation is that you hold off on this

# Basic customization

Now you're going to want to move through the customization of the blog, in which case you want to go down to the Personalize section and click on the theme button

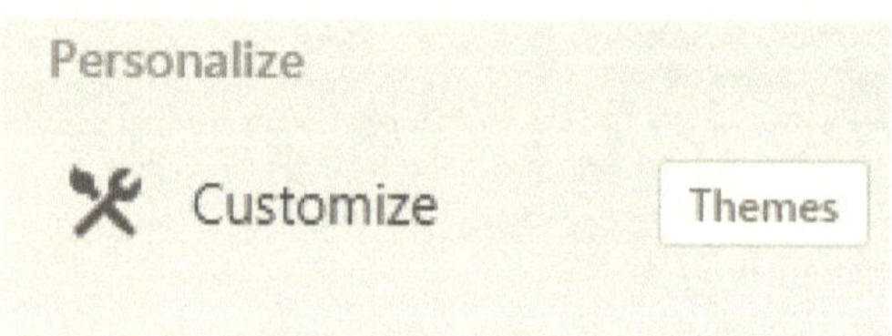


Picking a theme is probably one of the most fun things you can do, so take your time, and make sure you filter by only the Free themes for now and pick one that you love! Later on we will get to how to choose a proper paid theme.

After you've chosen your theme you'll want to click on the Customize button so that you can move through all the various elements that Wordpress.com allows you to do with just the Free plan. Many of these customizations are truly subjective, so it's entirely up to you on what you pick for the many different options. I will highlight below some of the very important things that must be in place from the beginning.

# Email Widget

A habit you will need to get into from the start is to start an email list for people to subscribe to your blog posts. This is a critical strategy for creating reader retention. If we manage to get someone to actually come to our blog and read our content, we want to do everything in our power to keep them coming back. More on this later. For now make sure you add the MailChimp Subscriper Popup widget to your site and test that it works.

Add a Widget

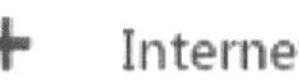

Displays an image.

Instagram

Display your latest Instagram photos.

Internet Defense League

Show your support for the Internet Defense League.

Links

Your blogroll

MailChimp Subscriber Popup

Allows displaying a popup subscription form to visitors.

Once added, click on the widget and then click the small help question mark next to "Code:". This opens the help page that walks you through how to create your MailChimp account and set up the popup form code to work on your site. Again, make sure you take the time to understand how MailChimp works and that your popup works properly because this will be critical going forward. Many bloggers make the mistake of not taking their email list serious from the beginning and pay the price for it later.

## Social Media Widget

You were probably wondering how far you could get into this Ebook before I mentioned Social Media. Well here we are. As I'm sure you may already be aware, social media is a critical component of distributing your content and driving reader loyalty and retention. I definitely recommend that you create accounts for your blog on the following platforms:

- Facebook Page
- Instagram
- Twitter
- Pinterest

Once you've created these accounts, make sure you add the social icons widget to your blog and each of those accounts as their own icon. These icons won't be a huge way in which you gain traction on social media, we will get into those strategies later, but here in the beginning it will absolutely help.

# GAINING INITIAL TRAFFIC

In this article I'll talk about some of the strategies that we used and thought were successful in getting views after we initially created the site. So let's take a look at what our traffic looked like:

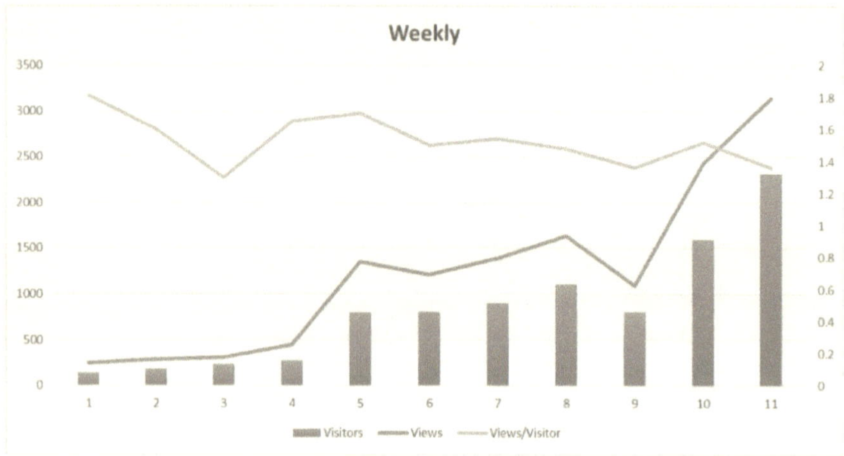


This is a weekly view of how our traffic progressed in the first 11 weeks. A couple of important things to note, look at how slow our traffic was in the first 4 weeks! **Do not be discouraged!** Building traffic on a website is a slow grind, but there are many strategies you can implement early that you will benefit from greatly in the long-run. Here are our strategies for the early game, right when your website is brand new.

## Wordpress Reader

If you've started out on Wordpress.com, then you can take advantage of a fantastic feature on the platform called the Wordpress Reader. The reader is a feed of article topics that you can actively subscribe to and thereby get a feed of articles that you are interested in. What this means for us is that there is a huge community of fellow beauty bloggers that you can put your articles in front of, entirely for free. There are some interesting quirks with this reader that allows us to drive a solid amount of traffic with little effort. The reader works through the various tags that a person places on their posts. This is done in that right sidebar under the categories section. The reader loads these articles entirely in chronological order and puts almost no emphasis but here are some important things to keep in mind.

- Use Tags - Use tags such as Makeup, Cosmetics, Beauty Blogger, Beauty, etc. but don't use too many. I believe the general advice is to use about 7-8.
- Actionable Titles - Make sure your title compels people to actually click! Make it interesting!
- Interesting Pictures - Important to make sure your featured image is a great one because that's the picture that will appear in the reader.
- Get Involved - Follow other blogs, like their articles, comment, etc. Many bloggers will follow back, and check out your articles if you do so on theirs. You'll notice when you post articles with proper tags that your articles will start getting comments, there's a reason they do this!

# TAKING THE NEXT STEP

Once you feel that you've exhausted the time as a free Wordpress.com blog and you are ready to take the next step, you have a choice you can make. You can either take a small step, and simply upgrade to the Wordpress.com first paid package. This package allows you to get a custom domain, it also provides a few more customization options. For ~$5 a month this is not a terrible deal for you to provide you relevance on the various search engines and to get your feet wet in the more advanced features of the Wordpress platform. If you choose to take this step, simply purchase a domain from one of the many domain providers, Namecheap is a good one. Once it is purchased then Wordpress walks you through the process of mapping the domain which is very straight forward.

The other option you have is to take the leap to the advanced hosting platforms. This will be about the same price but will involve you having to migrate all your content to a new host. The benefit here is that this is where you'll likely be for the rest of time with your website. All the features you could want are now available, it only requires a bit more effort on your part.

## Moving to Bluehost

Our recommendation is to go with a highly rated, very reliable host like Bluehost. I'll walk throughout this course not just of the benefits from choosing them, but also how you actually get your blog established.

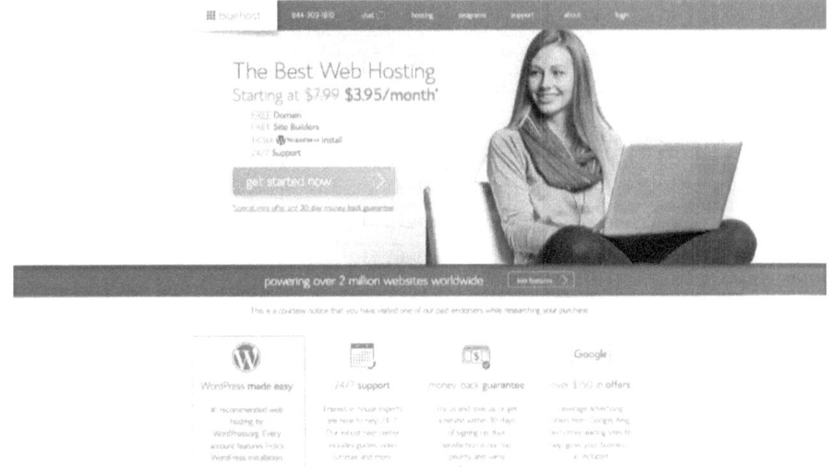

# Why start your Makeup Blog on Bluehost?

There is a reason Bluehost is so well regarded in the blogging community. Many top bloggers all recommend their platform for the simple reason its got all the significant benefits that will make your life extremely easy, rather than having to go through the pain of managing many of the grievances that come with actually making sure the website is functioning properly.

## Benefits for your Beauty Blog

The Bluehost pricing is really incredible. The basic plan comes with a ton of the features that you need if you want to keep things at their bare bones. However, if you upgrade for only an additional $2 per month you can get a whole HOST (no pun intended) of amazing additional benefits. I'll try to explain below why so many of these are awesome

- **Bandwidth** - Unmetered bandwidth is critical because you want to make sure if your site gets a big spike in traffic that you don't suddenly get a huge spike in price! You'll be paying the same amount each month regardless of the traffic level which can help you sleep at night knowing you won't get some huge bill suddenly.

- **SpamExperts** - Your blog will get a ton of spam, I'm warning you right now. The comment sections will be filled with random garbage and sorting through it all is a huge pain. Their SpamExperts really allow you to not waste your precious time cleaning up the spam and rather having that handled by people who truly know what they are doing. Spend more time blogging, not cleaning up spam!

- **Domain Privacy** - This is a great feature in that it allows the details around your domain registration to remain anonymous. You'd be surprised at how many weirdos are out there and having this piece of mind is great.

- **SiteBakeup Pro** - Having consistent high performance backups is critical. You never know what might happen and being able to restore your site from a backup will save your butt more times than you would think. If you attempt to manage this on your own you can find yourself in a lot of trouble and end up losing so much of what you've worked so hard on. Don't be one of those people, make sure your site is properly backed up.

- **Domain Management** - Bluehost also manages everything related to your site under one roof. You can map your domain to your site easily from their platform, rather than having to hop between 3 different platforms just to manage your domain.

Thank you for choosing Bluehost. You have made the right choice in selecting us as your web hosting and eBusiness provider. We provide excellent customer service, reliable hardware and affordable prices.

We appreciate your business and look forward to a great relationship.

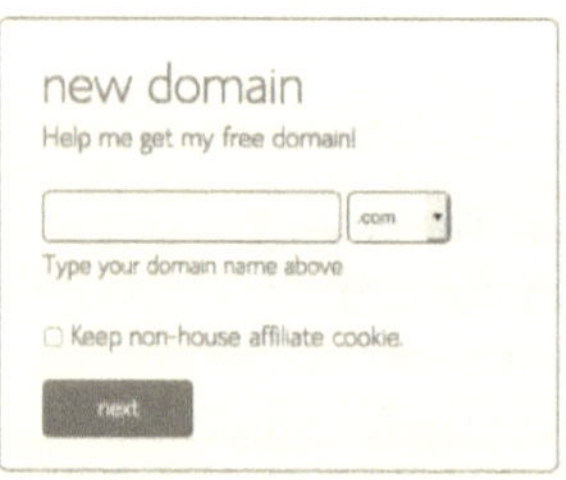


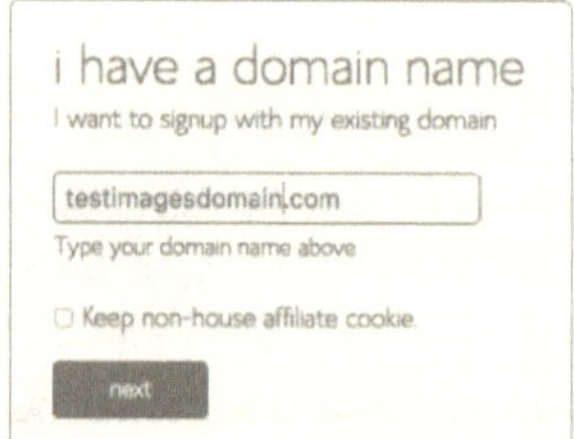


- **Wordpress Themes** - This is probably the second hardest thing you'll need to do, simply because it's so much fun! Bluehost also includes themes for you to choose and it's awesome to browse through to find the one that is perfect for you.

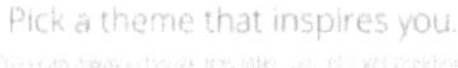

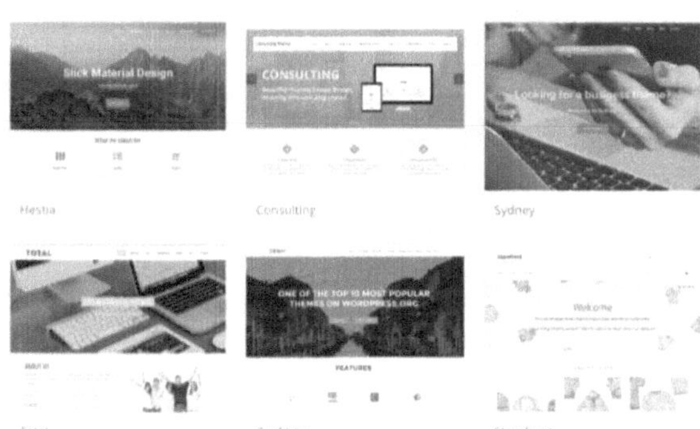

# How to Start

First to get started, head over to Bluehost. There you'll want to click the link for Get Started Now and then select your plan.

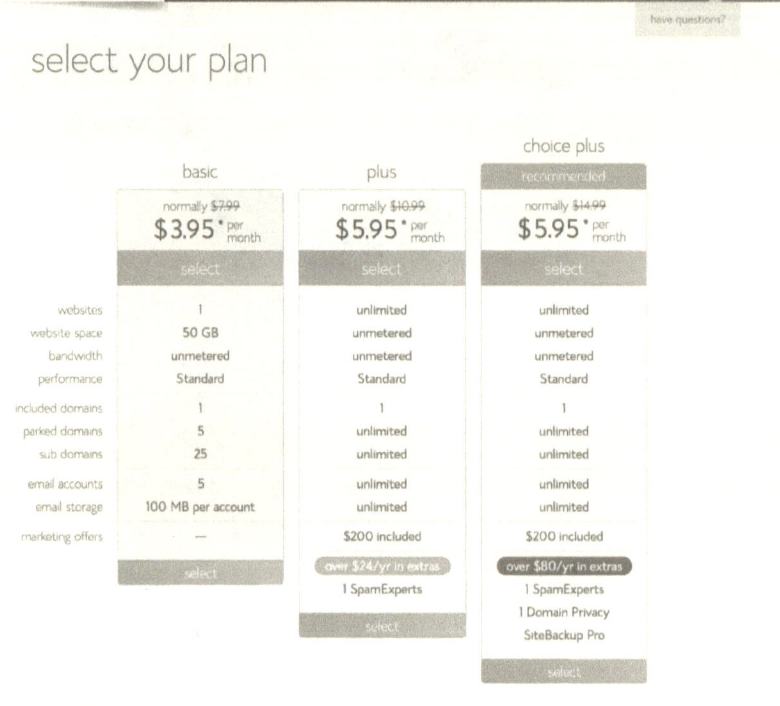

account information

All fields are required unless otherwise noted.

First Name

Last Name

(optional) Business Name

Country: United States

Street Address

City

State: Please select a state

ZIP Code

Phone Number: (123) 456-7890   Ext

Use an international number

*Email Address

*Your receipt will be sent to this address

package information

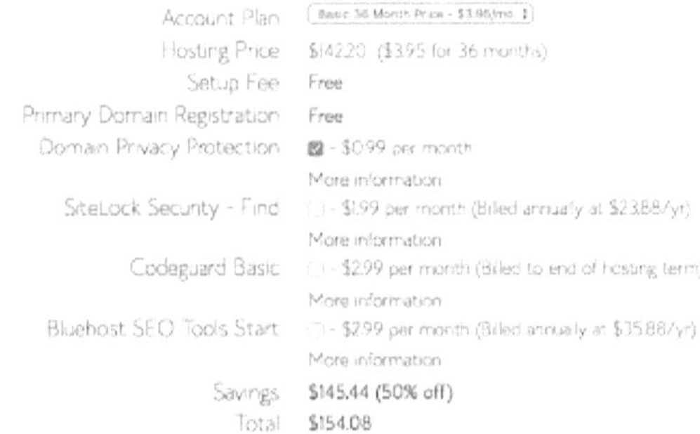


You'll typically save more money by singing up for yearly plans, so we definitely recommend doing that. You'll be asked to create a password for your account. Make sure you do a strong password here, you'll have a lot of hackers out there attempting to guess your password to mess with your site, so be sure it's a good one.

Choose a password for your account

Before you can login to your account or use your new hosting features, you first need to create a secure password - Please note this password and your hosting payment information, as these are used for account verification purposes when contacting Bluehost support.

Create your password

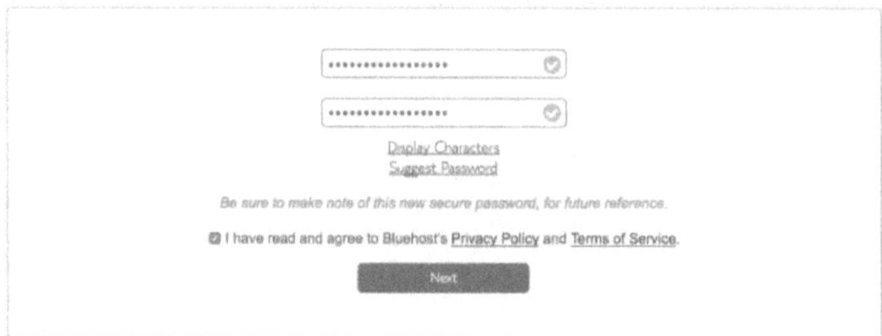


Next step will be to get a domain or map an existing domain to your website.



Now all you have to do now is choose a theme a theme or import your previous one.

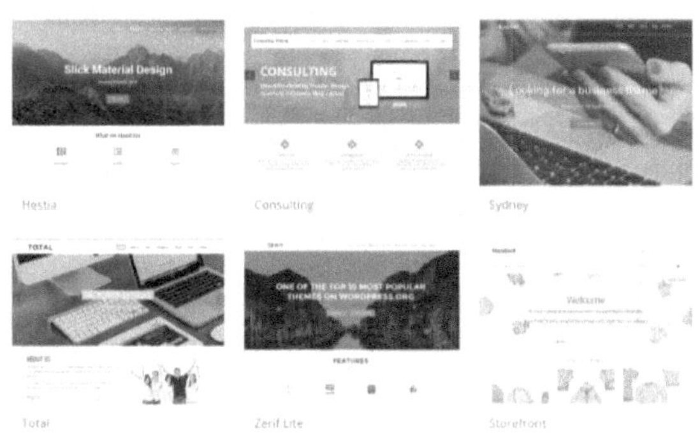



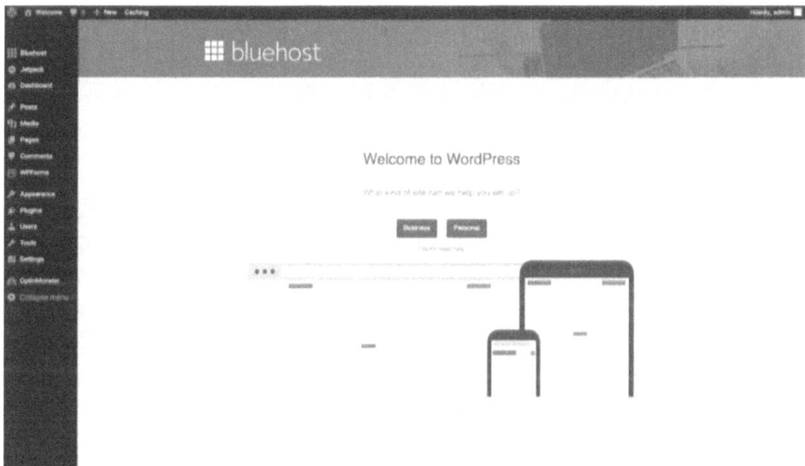



You are now ready to go!

# CREATING CONTENT AND FINDING YOUR VOICE – SOME ADVICE

At this point your blog should be up and running, fully customized utilizing all the features available under the free plan. Now all that's left to do is that you begin creating your content. Here is where I can only offer advice to help you shape your thinking around what you want you blog to be and what the vision for your creative process will be.

## *Comparison is the Thief of Joy*

I believe one of the best ways to become a creator of amazing content is to be a veracious consumer of said content. One of the best mindsets that I believe you can have when it comes to finding your voice is simply "Create the content that you would want to read." What is meant by this is that if you were creating blog posts or videos about makeup for a single persons enjoyment (that person being yourself) what type of content would you make? What would you enjoy reading? What interesting looks or topics do you find yourself really wanting content around? This may seem like such a no brainer, but you would be surprised at the amount of people who begin their journey with this mindset, but lose it once they get on the grind of becoming popular. Suddenly their vision isn't around what they enjoy making, it becomes, well what do people want to read? What's "in" right now? What are all the popular videos about? What are the top blog posts about? Oh that's the stuff I should be making! I'll explain my thinking around why I think this is wrong, and sticking to your roots will keep you sane.

They say that comparison is the thief of joy, and nowhere is that more evident than in the rat race to become a popular blogger in the beauty space. I've lost track of how many different makeup vloggers I've seen post long rants on their Youtube channels talking about how they are frustrated by their lack of growth. Even my own wife fell for this line of thinking and I've had to 'talk her off the ledge' multiple times and explain why it's an entirely flawed way to think about blogging and vlogging in general. Typically the thinking will start by them seeing a Blogger or Youtuber who has reached fantastic success in some small time frame, typically 1-2 years. Anyone looking at that situation will think to themselves, wow, how is it that someone can gain 300k subscribers in 2 years, yet I'm sitting at 500 after one year? Let me explain to you why that is not only normal, but guaranteed to be the case. The simple explanation is luck. You may not want to hear that but let me lay it out. If you look at the entirety of the makeup blogger cohort, there has to be thousands and thousands of them in total. Many people (yourself included) have decided to hop on the bandwagon and give it a try. Of those many thousands, you can naturally expect that some tiny percentage is going to get extraordinarily lucky and go viral, gaining a massive amount of popularity quickly. Perhaps this this individual is very talented or writes very well, that can absolutely be the case. However, so do many of the people who do not go viral. Many people are likely even more talented and produce even better content than these people, yet never hit that kind of meteoric success. What accounts for this? Entirely luck. What is happening here is that someone is looking at an individual who has essentially won the lottery, and then compares that to their own situation and starts to make the assessment that its due to *quality* differences or *the types of content* the person made that is the reason they went viral. I want to tell you and I hope you agree, this is just not true. These people have almost entirely gotten lucky. Since we cannot count on just winning the lottery to be successful, we will need to stick to the old faithful which is hard work and persistence. If you implement the proper strategies, and are constantly evaluating what you do to improve then with enough time I believe success can be achieved.

In that last sentence I emphasized that you need to provide "enough time" for things to unfold. Rome wasn't built in a day, and neither will your blogging empire. That is precisely why my advice is to create content that you genuinely enjoy making because if you start making content that is unenjoyable, then its going to be a slow and painful grind to the top. Many people cannot stand to do tedious writing for years on end. The going will be slow, so let's make sure it's fun!

## Be Unique (Sort of)

Now that you've settled on creating content that you love, the next thing that many people will inevitably say is, well there's already people writing about that topic! I need to be absolutely unique or else no one will read! This line of thinking is also not true, but it has hints of truth to it. My advice is to aim to be only sort of unique. Just because there's a Walgreens, doesn't mean that CVS can't exist. A practical example was for us, that even when our site was rather new we would write about certain products that had already been covered by some of the big blogs. They tended to dominate the top results, but guess who started appear right after them? We did. Over time we just starting bumping up against their rankings and in some cases would rank higher than them. If you make good content that has a new and entertaining or informative view, people are always interested in seeing alternative opinions or views so you can absolutely start to eat the lunch of your competition. By combining this mindset with the various SEO strategies, making sure to target quality long-tail keywords, will provide you that opportunity to carve out your slice of the pie.

# MONETIZING YOUR BLOG

You were probably wondering when we would get to the part about how to make some money. Well here I'll lay out the various avenues that you have in front of you. Some of these you will not be able to take advantage of from the beginning and it will depend on which stage your blog is in as to whether you can turn on this income stream. I'll put a note next to each one as to whether it's available for Beginners or Advanced, with the distinction being on whether you are hosting on Bluehost or still on Wordpress.com

## *Affiliate Marketing – Beginner*

Affiliate marketing is entering into a relationship with individual brands that if someone from your website clicks a link to the brands website and subsequently purchases something, then you get a commission on that sale. The commission percentage can vary greatly from anywhere as low as 0.68% to 25%. It will entirely depend on the individual affiliate programs and how you've joined them. The key to this one is to join as many programs as possible. Since the Makeup industry has so many different brands, you'll want to make sure you're already in a program with as many as possible just in case you end up writing about them in the future. It can often take quite a while to be accepted into programs so you do not want to wait until they are relevant to try to join. To join affiliate programs you will need to join various affiliate platforms. On these platforms is where the brands will be listed and you can apply to join their programs. Here is a list of all important affiliate programs you'll need to join:

- Amazon
- Linkshare
- Pepperjam

- Commission Junction
- Refersion
- ShareASale
- VigLink

In the appendix I've added our most up to date list of all makeup affiliate programs and on which platform they are located. The programs constantly shut down or move to other platforms so apologies if the list is not perfect.

When you are starting out affiliate programs can be kind of a pain because when you apply the brands will typically take a look at your site to make sure they want their brands promoted there. You will find yourself getting randomly rejected for no good reason. My suggestion is to first, don't let it get you down, and second, don't overplay your hand early. If you reapply constant to some brands programs they may blacklist you entirely. Therefore, if you get denied just move to the backup plan.

The backup plan is this wonderful affiliate platform called VigLink. VigLink is the affiliate platform of affiliate platforms. What they've done is that you essentially create an account with them, and they in turn are part of all these different affiliate programs, giving you instant access to virtually all of them. The downside here is that Viglink takes a cut of your commission. In the beginning this is a perfectly find price to pay since some programs (such as Sephora and Ulta) are unavailable to small bloggers. Once you are more established my suggestion is that you try to replace your VigLink affiliate links with the direct affiliate link once you are able to join all the individual brands programs on your own. VigLink is a stepping stone that you have to move off eventually.

Other than simply sharing the affiliate links of the products you are writing about, your goal should be to get coupon codes with as many brands as possible. We see a significant jump in conversions with brands where we have a coupon code with even a small discount attached. Reason being is that people will be more inclined to make the purchase as well as, you getting credit for the sale if your coupon code is used. There's always the chance that the person loses your affiliate cookie before making the purchase, so the coupon code saves you many times.

## Advertising – Advanced

Advertising on your blog using the big ad platforms such as Amazon and Google is only something you can take advantage of once you are hosted on a proper platform like Bluehost. Wordpress.com does not allow you to put the adcode on your site.

## Google Ads

The King of advertising is absolutely Google. The reason they've earned this spot is because they pay content creators the most out of any other and they make life super easy for us to install their ads. My suggestion is that after you make an Adsense account, you implement the Auto Ads. Auto Ads is a feature where Google will actually place the ads wherever it wants on your site without you having to designate exactly where the ads should show up and in what format. The reason I love this is because Google is actually very good at tastefully placing your ads. I've seen virtually no examples where the ad was placed in an obnoxious and ugly place on our site. You should definitely test this thoroughly to see if this is a good fit for you. Otherwise you can always create your own ad units and place them specifically on the site where you would like them to appear. Auto Ads is also great because it implements mobile ads which are some of the best performing units you can have.

To implement the Auto Ads is very easy. You simply configure which types of ads you want it to insert, then Google will provide you the code that you have to place in the Header of your theme code. Go to Appearance > Editor, then in the Theme files find your Theme Header. Then place the code that google provided anywhere between the <head> and </head> tag you'll see at the top.

## Amazon Recommended Ads

When you join Amazon's Affiliate program, you'll have the ability to create Amazon Recommended Ads. These ad units will show relevant products to your readers. These ads perform wonderfully and they are very easy to add as well.

Once you've walked through the process of choosing the features of your Amazon ads, you'll get ad code that you'll need to place on your blog in the spots where you want it to appear. Important to note here that you will have to create a new ad for every single spot on your page, so you can't just reuse the same one over and over. An ad code can only show an ad once per page, so if you want to show three separate Amazon Ads on one page or post, you'll have to create three separate ads.

## Sponsored Content – Advanced

Sponsored content is something I'd consider more of a mature blog opportunity rather than being exclusive to an advanced blog. The reason being is that the brands that will be paying you to write content are typically not interested in paying you unless your traffic and reach has gotten to a sufficient level. I believe the threshold for where sponsored content becomes relevant is around 40-50k page views per month. Prior to this stage you will have a very difficult time getting any attention from brands.

To get sponsored content opportunities you have two options in front of you. You can either try to contact brands directly or sign up for Sponsored Post platforms and apply for individual campaigns that are available. Similar to the affiliate programs, you'll need to join a number of different platforms to get access to all the opportunities. I'd suggest that you make accounts on the following platforms:

- https://www.tomoson.com/
- https://activate.bloglovin.com/
- https://influence.co/

As you browse these, specifically Influence.co, you'll see what brands are interested in and what types of reach and traffic is required to qualify for these campaigns.

## PR Packages and Free Products – Beginner

Fortunately, getting free products is something that you can take advantage of from almost the very beginning. Free products can come either organically from brands reaching out to you for reviews and unboxings. You'll likely see more indie brands doing this when you're new but even at lower levels of traffic you may get contacted by legitimate brands as well. The agreement usually is that if they send you the products then you need to do a comprehensive review of them. It's important to note that the reviews don't have to be positive, they just need to be fair. Many bloggers will feel pressured to provide a positive review but don't entertain it. It's important that you do include the disclosure that the product was provided for free to ensure that you are complaint with FTC guidelines (assuming you are in the US).

The other option is to contact brands directly. Try to locate a good email address of something who is likely able to actually provide you the products. In other words, don't just email their customer service. The more people between you and the free product person, the harder it will be. A great source of these direct contacts is through the affiliate programs. Each affiliate program usually has an affiliate manager listed in the details of the program. We've had solid success in talking to this person and actually getting a decision made on whether they will send us products. The template we use for these emails is pasted here:

Hello,

We run Makeupfomo.com and we are part of your affiliate program on _______. We wanted to hear if it would be possible to receive some products for review? We believe a well written review and video of your products would resonate with our audience. Also, we've seen a lot of success with other brands with getting a custom coupon code to share with our readers. Ideally this would be MAKEUPFOMO giving a small discount off a purchase.

Coupon codes and product reviews will be shared on the following platforms:

- Makeupfomo.com - ___k+ page views per month, ___% CTR
- Email list - _____ email subscribers, ___% open rate, ___% CTR
- Youtube Channel - ___ subscribers
- Instagram - ___ followers

Examples of other product reviews:

- http://makeupfomo.com/2017/05/25/karity-unicorn-dreams-eyeshadow-palette/
- http://makeupfomo.com/2017/01/12/karity-just-peachy-eyeshadow-palette/
- http://makeupfomo.com/2018/06/18/kviiiln-genie-glow-highlighters-review/
- http://makeupfomo.com/2018/07/16/pur-sweet-sixteen-collection/

Let me know if any of the above would be possible. Thank you!

Running this strategy is good when you are a low-to-medium sized blog (0-50k pageviews per month). Once you get into the 50K page views range, it's time to create a proper media kit with much more extensive information about various promotional opportunities brands can have with you.

# DISTRIBUTION STRATEGY

The distribution strategy is all about how you get your content in front of as many eyeballs as possible. The critical piece that people often miss is that this is the most important piece and where so much of your thinking and focus needs to be. The specific strategy that you end up settling into is going to depend entirely on your blog. This is going to need to be fine-tuned to the specific DNA of how your blog operates, the type of content you make, the type of audience you tend to attract, and those various factors. That being said, there are some fundamental ways in which you approach distribution which I will outline. Once you get into it you will start to notice what specific ideas are working best and start to ramp up or ramp down your effort into each. I think it's critical to take a scientific view point to this. You are running experiments on your blog continuously to learn what works best and what does not work. This is another element that many bloggers (me included) really kick themselves that they didn't get into from an early stage and are only attempting to catch up late into the game.

## Setting up Experiments

The elements needed to run these experiments is very simply, but it's the discipline and persistence to apply it constantly to make sure you can collect the dividends that this strategy provides. First thing you need to do is to create a Google Analytics account and to add the tag ID to your website (mind you that you cannot do this within the Wordpress.com lower price and free packages). This is something you can only do once you are on a proper hosting platform. You will still be able to pull through the important stats on the free hosting, however it has a tendency to be unreliable in my opinion. Although it's unreliable, it still adds value for you to understand which experiments are providing positive results.

The basic structure of these experiments is that you will add specific source tags to the links that you send to various platforms (Facebook, twitter, Instagram, Pinterest) that give you detailed information about where the person clicked the link and came to your website. A basic way to do this is to add the following code to the end of any link /?utm_source=ANYTHINGHERE. So an example of this would be https://makeupfomo.com/?utm_source=EbookLink. You can use googles URL builder to help you with this: https://ga-dev-tools.appspot.com/campaign-url-builder/.

This tool allows you to easily add campaign parameters to URLs so you can track Custom Campaigns in C Analytics.

Enter the website URL and campaign information

Fill out the required fields (marked with *) in the form below, and once complete the full campaign URL v generated for you. *Note: the generated URL is automatically updated as you make changes.*

| | |
|---|---|
| * Website URL | http://makeupfomo.com |
| | The full website URL (e.g. `https://www.example.com`) |
| * Campaign Source | Calendar |
| | The referrer: (e.g. `google`, `newsletter`) |
| Campaign Medium | |
| | Marketing medium: (e.g. `cpc`, `banner`, `email`) |

What this will do is that when a person clicks on the link, it will pass through the utm_source value EbookLink to your analytics screen and it will bucket those visitors by themselves. So what you can end up doing is that if you have an idea to distribute your blogs on twitter using a specific hashtag, then the link you put on twitter should have the source tag as something like TwitterHashtag1. That way you can monitor over time whether that strategy actually led to people coming to the site.

Practical example of this implemented: In the beginning I was distributing our blog posts onto Google+ and their various boards. These boards are free to join and in many cases have tens of thousands of people in them, so I figured this would be an awesome place to add our blog posts. I added the ?utm_source=GooglePlusBoards to the links that I put on these boards and over a few weeks I spent a good amount of time adding our posts to the many different relevant boards. And what would you guess my experiment told me? Almost zero traffic. I figured out that although these boards have so many followers, there was practically zero engagement. People just didn't click on the links, and when they did, they spent almost no time on my site making their traffic worthless for our purposes. My conclusion after this experiment was pretty simply. I wouldn't waste any more time posting to Google+. This was a pretty straight forward example, however the same type of thinking can be applied to try to maximize the traffic and engagement you get from different channels. As with any experiment, you want to go into it with a solid hypothesis as to what you think the result will be, what you need to see in order to learn that your guess was correct, and your next steps based on whether or not that ends up being correct or not. The important thing is to constantly iterate through this process with the goal being to consistently increase performance. Remember that you also need to allow these experiments enough time to give you meaningful data.

# DISTRIBUTION CHANNELS

*Reddit*

If you've never heard of Reddit before, I'd suggest you pop over to Reddit.com and take a look. Reddit is one of the largest websites on the internet and is a place where people can share interesting content about literally anything you can think of. Posting your blog posts here is a very delicate process because since Reddit is such a massive community, the moderators of the various Subreddits (the individual communities) are hyper aware of anyone attempting to drive traffic to their blog by sharing their links. Therefore it's often very likely that your posts will be deleted outright or your account will be banned if you attempt to do so. As such there are really two approaches you can take if you want to be able to tap into Reddit as a source for traffic.

The first method is to carefully insert your links into discussions where it is very relevant or to submit your links as part of a free content package for the subreddit. Essentially this requires that you write up a substantial amount of information, submit it to a subreddit either as it's own self-post or in the comments where the conclusion of your post or comment has a link to your blog post. If you browse many subreddits you'll see this used quite often, /r/entrepreneur is a common one. In my humble opinion this is a tough gig. Often it can be difficult to even find discussions or topics relevant enough that it'll catch the interest of the community as well as actually making the post or comment relevant enough to not get flagged as blog spam. I personally do not use this approach, but if you can make it work it can be an enormous source of traffic.

The second method is to simply make your own subreddit for your blog. Anyone can create a subreddit which is to make a community that people can subscribe to. Then you simply start adding posts to this subreddit and wait for people to naturally subscribe on their own. This is a very slow but low effort approach that can really pay off for two reasons. One reason is that Reddit sometimes ranks really nicely on search engines and will actually allow you to drive traffic despite your actual website ranking fairly low. So instead of people seeing your link when they google, they will see the post on Reddit, go there, then click the link to your site (remember your experiments!). Second, if you get lucky and a community begins to develop, people who are subscribed will see your posts appear in their feed on Reddit so you have that awesome retention we desperately are looking for.

## Facebook Page

Creating a Facebook Page almost goes without saying. I won't spend much time here to explain why this is absolutely necessary because the reasons should be obvious to most. This is a fantastic channel for creating reader retention, for pushing your content to new readers (i.e. someone likes your post, it may show up in their friends newsfeed, now you've got new readers), as well as, making it easy for people to share your content further on facebook. Many blogs see substantial amounts of traffic from Facebook alone so make sure you jump on the bandwagon of encouraging your readers to like your Facebook page.

## Instagram

I have a love/hate relationship with Instagram. I love it because it's a fairly easy set and forget channel to manage. I hate it because it feels almost entirely useless for anything other than vanity until you grow a substantial following, but even then I have my doubts. My reasons for finding Instagram useless is that you will drive close to zero traffic from the platform. That link in your bio is rarely clicked so as far as actually driving traffic, you will really not see it from there. The same goes for the links in stories. In our experience from being featured on a few brands Instagram stories with direct swipe up links to the site, we saw virtually no traffic from being featured. Maybe we got unlucky, but this definitely did not make me hate Instagram less. The main reason you need Instagram is to "prove" to the world that you are important. Brands and advertisers look to your follower count to access how popular you are and how much engagement you are able to drive. Many advertising and sponsored content campaigns require Instagram posts and stories, so the amount of followers you will be showing this to is very important. So if the people holding the money say they want big Instagram numbers, well then we are just going to need to get some big Instagram numbers.

To manage Instagram is very easy. There are some fantastic services that allow you to easily schedule and manage everything on Instagram so you can sit back and let it do the work. Later.gg allows you to schedule up to 30 posts per month for free with one account which is more than enough for someone starting out. Obviously the important thing here is to make sure that you do research on the hashtags that are popular in your specific niche. To research this just head to the explore tab and look at what is showing up, really take note of the types of pictures and hashtags that are making it to your explore tab because that is what you need to target to get into other's explore tab. Make sure you take high quality pictures, do some research on how to take great pictures with proper composition and lighting and then schedule a post to go up almost every single day. As with many of these distribution channels the key is to be consistent. Post as often as you can, and post good quality content.

## *Pinterest*

Pinterest is the absolute queen in the beauty / makeup niche. This is your opportunity to dominate. If Pinterest does not end up being one of your top sources of traffic then you know you are not doing what you could be. The beauty (pun intended) about Pinterest is that it has this natural way that your posts can go absolutely viral and continue to go viral for ages to come. To take advantage of this youll have to make sure that you create a business account on Pinterest. You do this by creating a regular account, then upgrade it for free to business. Then you'll have to claim your website which involves simply adding a tag to your site that Pinterest provides. It usually takes a day or two before your website is officially claimed.

The strategy: Much like Instagram, a continuous source of great quality pictures is imperative here. I advise you to get in the habit that any time you make a new blog post or do anything in your life related to your niche, take tons of pictures. Even if the pictures aren't fantastic, you'll want to add all of these to Pinterest. My strategy that has proven to work is to simply "spray and pray". You upload tons of pins that are all highly keyword optimized to boards that are also highly optimized and then just hoping some of them gain traction. The benefit from this strategy is that you don't end up spending ridiculous amounts of time creating these perfect infographic pins that ultimately could end up not going viral at all. I've attempted to use this ach in the past and based on my experiments (this is why they are so important) I was able to see that it was not worth the effort to create these elaborate infographs. Great pictures of relevant things (eyeshadow palettes, products, makeup looks, designs) with the right keyword and pin optimization can go further than a single pin or two that you spent 2 hours on to create.

Pin optimization has to do with making sure that Pinterest ranks your pictures high when someone searches. Pinterest is like any other search engine. It looks for what it thinks is relevant to what the person searched, and brings that high in the results for them. So how does Pinterest decide what is relevant and what isn't? Well based on my experiments there are a number of places that seem to make a big difference. Pin description, Image file name, board name, and board description. What you will want to do with each of these four is that you make sure that you pepper them with the keywords you are attempting to target. The way to find the relevant keywords is to do some searching for high level words relevant to your content. If you're writing about eyeshadows, you can search in the Pinterest bar and see what relevant search terms show up.

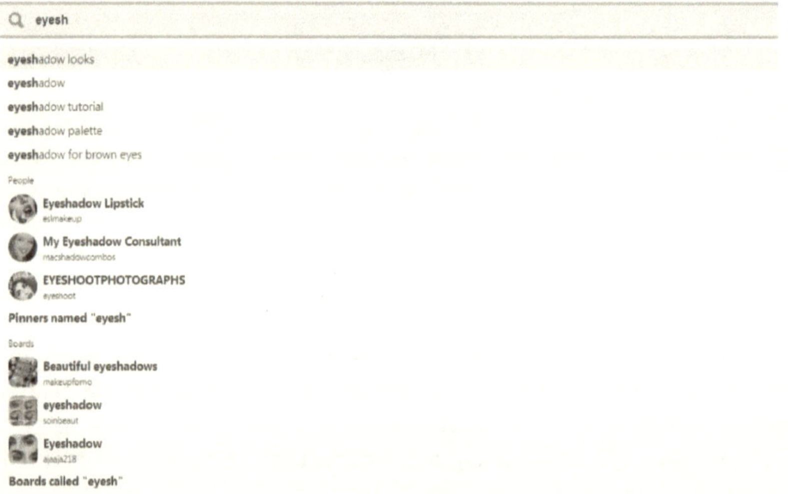


Some of them could be Eyeshadow looks, eyeshadow looks for brown eyes, eyeshadow guide step by step, etc. So now that you know Pinterest is indicating to you that these are the words people typically search by, you'll want to incorporate these into the various elements I listed above. The way to do this for the eyeshadow example would be: make the description for the pin: "Such a pretty **eyeshadow look**, this **tutorial** will give you the **eyeshadow guide** on how to go **step by step** to create a **makeup look** for **summer or fall fashion**... etc" You see what I did there right? I tried to naturally incorporate as many long-tail keywords into the description while making a coherent sentence. You want to do the same even for the image file name. Just name that thing "Eyeshadow palette look tutorial guide etc etc.jpg" before you upload it to Pinterest. Follow this same approach for your boards as well as the URLs to your blog posts.

## Twitter

Twitter is another platform that I'm not particular excited about but is very easy to set and forget that you may as well just do it. Once you've created your twitter account, make sure that you have the Jetpack widget installed on your site and link your twitter account to it. That way it'll automatically share your posts to Twitter and you don't have to think twice about it. We haven't had too much luck driving good traffic from it, perhaps you can crack the nut on this one. Otherwise I wouldn't waste too much time and energy on it if it doesn't work.

## Search Engine Optimization

SEO is a topic that there is just so much incredible content available for free that I won't waste time trying to replicate it in this Ebook. Here are a number of links that you should go through to understand how to optimize your pages and posts to give yourself the best chance to rank on Google, Bing, and the rest. The strategy is very similar to what I described in the Pinterest section. Focus on long tail keywords and be very consistent from the beginning. Here are the links that are a must read:

- On Page SEO - https://neilpatel.com/blog/the-on-page-seo-cheat-sheet/
- Everything SEO related - https://neilpatel.com/blog/

# CLOSING THOUGHTS AND NEXT STEPS

The hope is that this book can give you the details and strategies to get out there into the blogging world and grow your blog to a sufficient level. In an effort from keeping this book to become obnoxiously long, I've also created a Udemy course where I detail the in-depth configuration and set up of a Wordpress blog on other hosting platforms such as Amazon Lightsail, all the important plugins that I recommend over the long term, how to implement SSL, automated and advanced ways to distribute to the various channels. If you are feel that you are ready to take the Masterclass on how to create your successful Makeup blog, you can head over to Udemy and find my course: How To Start a Successful Makeupp & Beauty Blog Masterclass and use coupon code EBOOKEXCLUSIVE for 50% off.

# LIST OF AFFILIATE PROGRAMS

**Brand Name     Affiliate Program**

- 100% Pure          Shareasale
- Ace Beaute          Their Own
- Adept     Refersion
- AHAVA    Linkshare
- All Beauty           VigLink
- Amore Pacific      Linkshare
- Antonym Cosmetics          Shareasale
- Athena Cosmetics / revitalash cosmetics       Commission Junction
- Au Naturale Cosmetics         Shareasale
- Avene USA           Linkshare
- Avon      VigLink
- Ayla        Shareasale
- Baby Quasar        Linkshare
- Bardou    Linkshare
- Bare Minerals       Pepperjam
- Be Pure Beauty     Refersion
- Beauty Bakerie     Impact Radius
- Beauty Brands      Linkshare
- Beauty Bridge      Linkshare
- Beauty Care Choices          Pepperjam
- Beauty Con          Pepperjam
- Beauty Encounter VigLink
- Beauty Plus Salon Linkshare
- Beauty Trends      VigLink

- Beautylish       Shareasale
- Bella Cuore      Refersion
- Bellacie  Refersion
- Benefit   VigLink
- Besame Cosmetics       Shareasale
- BH Cosmetics    Linkshare
- Black Opal       VigLink
- Blissworld       VigLink
- Bobbi Brown Cosmetics    VigLink
- Borderlinx       Linkshare
- Bubble T Cosmetics       VigLink
- BurberryVigLink
- Butter London    Shareasale
- Buxom   Linkshare
- Camomile        Shareasale
- Candy Lipz       Commission Junction
- Cargo Cosmetics  Pepperjam
- Carols Daughter  VigLink
- Charlotte Tilbury VigLink
- Chic allue       Refersion
- Chrislie  Pepperjam
- Ciate London    Their Own
- Civilized Cosmetics      Pepperjam
- Clarria Cosmetics VigLink
- Clinique Linkshare
- Coastal Scents    Shareasale
- Colleen Rothschild Beauty Linkshare
- Concrete Minerals       Pepperjam
- Cosmetic AmericaLinkshare
- Crown Brush     Their Own
- Cult Beauty      VigLink
- Cuvee Beauty    Shareasale
- D Benoit Cosmetics       Their Own
- Deco Miami Cosmetics     VigLink
- Decorte  Pepperjam
- Derma Doctor    Linkshare
- Dermelect       Pepperjam
- DHC Beauty      Linkshare
- e.l.f.     Linkshare

- Ecco Bella        Shareasale
- Elizabeth Arden   VigLink
- Espionage         Refersion
- Esque    Refersion
- Estee Lauder UK   Linkshare
- Estee Lauder US   Linkshare
- Eve Organics      Refersion
- Fabriah  VigLink
- Farmacy Skincare Shareasale
- First Aid Beauty   Commission Junction
- Fitglow Beauty    Shareasale
- Flower Beauty     Shareasale
- Fountain Cosmetics        Viglink
- Furless Cosmetics Their Own
- Gabriel Cosmetics Shareasale
- Gerard Cosmetics Pepperjam
- Giorgio Armani Beauty     VigLink
- Girlactik Cosmetics       Shareasale
- Glossier  Linkshare
- Glow Cult         Refersion
- Grande Cosmetics Pepperjam
- H20+     Pepperjam
- Habit Cosmetics   Refersion
- Happy Farm Botanicals     Linkshare
- Harrods  VigLink
- Hourglass         VigLink
- Illamasqua        Affilinet
- IT Cosmetics      VigLink
- J Nicole Skincare  Pepperjam
- Jacqueline Deviante       Their Own
- Jane Affiliates    Shareasale
- Johnny Concert   VigLink
- jolie beauty      Pepperjam
- Josie Maran       Pepperjam
- Jouer    Linkconnector
- Juice Beauty       Linkshare
- Julep     Shareasale
- June Jacobs       Linkshare
- Kaleidoscope      Refersion

- Kali Beauty        Pepperjam
- Kaplan MD Skincare        Linkshare
- Karity    Shareasale
- Kat Von D        Linkshare
- Kate Somerville    Pepperjam
- Katherine Cosmetics        Pepperjam
- Kiko Milano        Pepperjam
- Kiss and Makeup  Shareasale
- Klorane  Linkshare
- Koh Gen Do        Linkshare
- Kohgendo        VigLink
- LA Splash Cosmetics        Their own
- Labelle Makeup   Their Own
- Lancome        Flexoffers
- Laneige  Linkshare
- LAQA & Co        Shareasale
- Laura Geller Beauty        Linkshare
- Laura Mercier    Linkshare
- Laxmi    Shareasale
- Leaders Cosmetics        Shareasale
- Lena Lashes        Affiliatly
- Lilah B.  Pepperjam
- Lilumia  Linkshare
- Lime Crime        Commission Junction
- LipLand  Their Own
- Liz Early Linkshare
- Lord & Taylor    Linkshare
- Love Lula        Pepperjam
- lucious  Refersion
- Luxie Beauty    Their Own
- MAC Cosmetics (Estee)    Emailed them
- Makeup Geek    Their Own
- Marc Jacobs    VigLink
- MD-Factor    Linkshare
- Mellow Cosmetics        VigLink
- MemeBox        Linkshare
- Michael Todd Beauty        Linkshare
- Milk Makeup    Linkshare
- Molly Cosmetics  Refersion

- Mommy Makeup  Shareasale
- MyChelle Dermaceudicals  Linkshare
- NA-KD   Linkshare
- NARS     Pepperjam
- Naturally Better You        Linkshare
- OFRA     https://www.ofracosmetics.com/pages/affiliates
- Ole Henriksen     Linkshare
- Omorovicza     Linkshare
- Outer Beauty Cosmetics    Linkshare
- OZ Naturals     Linkshare
- Pat McGrath Labs Pepperjam
- Percy & Reed Product     Linkshare
- Peridot   Refersion
- Peter Thomas Roth        Linkshare
- Philosophy USA   Commission Junction
- Pixi Beauty        Shareasale
- Planet Beauty       Shareasale
- PLAZAN Cosmetics          Shareasale
- PUR      Commission Junction
- Pur~lisse        Pepperjam
- Real Her Shareasale
- Sally Beauty       VigLink
- Saucebox        Refersion
- Sephora  Viglink
- Shany Cosmetics  Linkshare
- Sigma Beauty       VigLink
- Sleek Studio      Their Own
- Smashbox       VigLink
- Smashbox UK     Linkshare
- Soko Glam        Pepperjam
- Stila cosmetics    VigLink
- Stowaway Cosmetics       Commission Junction
- Sulwhasoo       Linkshare
- Tarte Cosmetics  Pepperjam
- Tatcha   VigLink
- Tempty  Linkshare
- Too Faced        Impact Radius
- Treat Beauty       Shareasale
- Ulta       VigLink

- Urban Decay	Viglink
- Urban Decay Canada	Pepperjam
- Vanatei	Refersion
- Vanity Planet	Linkshare
- Vera Mona	Refersion
- Violet Voss	Refersion
- Void Beauty	VigLink
- WEI EastLinkshare
- Yves Rocher	Commission Junction
- Zest Beauty	VigLink